I0696814

FIX YOUR FITNESS

Achieve Boundless Energy.
Unleashing the Power of Fitness
for a Vibrant Life

By

Norman G. Johns

DISCLAIMER

Table of Contents

Introduction:

Are you ready to reclaim your life and experience the transformative power of fitness?

Are you capable of embracing fitness for total wellness—mind and body—and empowering yourself?

Maintaining a good level of physical fitness is vitally important. However, it could be difficult to define what fitness entails. Several physical health issues can influence one's level of physical fitness.

According to experts, physical fitness refers to "one's capacity to carry out daily activities with while managing disease, weariness, and stress and reducing sedentary behavior, one should strive for optimum efficiency, strength, and endurance.

"

This encompasses more than just being able to run quickly or carry a ton of weight. Despite being significant

How physically fit someone is depends on how well they meet each of the criteria for being healthy.

We have spent our entire lives hearing the words "health" and "fitness." By employing phrases like "health is wealth" and "fitness is the key," we are putting it into practice.

What does the word "health" actually mean? It refers to the idea of "being well." We refer to someone as being healthy and fit when they are in good bodily and mental health.

It's crucial to always keep in mind that we cannot maintain outstanding health and fitness on our own. Both the physical environment and the food's quality are important. Remember that our daily routines have an impact on our level of fitness. Our level of fitness is enhanced by the caliber of our diet, air, and water.

In Fix Your Fitness, we'll embark on a transformational journey together. It's time to let go of the limitations that have held us back and embrace a life full of grit, confidence, and vigor. By learning how to get fitter, we unlock the potential to succeed in all aspects of our lives.

So. Let's embark on this inspiring journey to realize our full potential.

Chapter 1

The Wake-up Call

If your early memories of gym class are ones of dread, shame, and failure, it may change how you view your own physical capabilities years later and may affect how likely you are to get off the couch as an adult.

A study found that persons who had negative gym memories as kids were less inclined to exercise as adults whereas those who had positive gym memories as kids were more likely to keep their fitness levels up. That is not surprising,

Although you cannot undo the past, you may alter your view on fitness.

You could think that working out requires a certain length of treadmill time, but assumptions of this sort can be problematic.

A fixed mindset, which focuses on whether you are intrinsically "good" at anything, is preferred to a growth mindset, which recognizes that development is possible even when learning something new is challenging. Instead of concentrating on the past, congratulate yourself on recommitting to a healthy lifestyle and acknowledging your accomplishments. Instead of focusing on the good feelings in your body, attempt to focus on them.

going to the gym frequently throughout the week is preferable to working out for two hours on the weekends.

A static ball is more challenging to move than one that is currently in motion, just like in physics. It takes consistency to break old habits. If you wait until you feel like working out, it could never happen. Additionally, if you only exercise sometimes, you run the risk of hurting yourself.

Try something new, like Zumba or a water class; work out while enjoying your favorite music, podcast, or TV show; go on a date with a friend; or exercise outside in a beautiful setting.

Simply put, everyone should exercise and be physically active. All ages of people, a kid, teenagers, or adults regular physical activity,   Physical activity promotes excellent health regardless of your body type or BMI, therefore you should stay active your entire life.

By being aware of the benefits of physical fitness and being aware of the right amount of activity, you may preserve excellent health and improve your general quality of life. Here are a few benefits of consistent exercise that highlight how important physical well-being is.

Save money; 7 out of 10 fatalities in the United States are attributed to chronic illnesses, which account for 86% of healthcare spending in the country, according to the Centers for Disease Control and Prevention. Even though some diseases cannot be prevented, you can reduce your risk for ailments like diabetes and heart disease by giving up risky habits and adopting a healthy lifestyle.

Making healthy choices, such as exercising frequently, can reduce your risk for several disorders and consequences that could require expensive medical care.

Increase your life expectancy: Numerous studies have shown that regular exercise increases longevity and decreases the risk of dying young. Although there isn't a magic formula that will turn physical activity into extra hours of life, research shows that more active people tend to be healthier and live longer.

Regular exercise lowers your chance of injury while enhancing bone density, flexibility, stability, and muscular strength. Being physically active can help you live a longer, healthier life by reducing your risk of accidental injuries and strengthening your body's defenses against them. For instance, if you have stronger muscles and better balance, you'll be less likely to trip and fall, and if you do, you'll be less likely to sustain bone injuries.

A sedentary lifestyle and a lack of exercise can be harmful to one's health. Improve your quality of life. Lack of exercise increases the risk of getting a number of chronic diseases, such as cancer, as well as a number of mental health issues. However, research has shown that in addition to its many other physical benefits, exercise has a favorable effect on mood and mental health. Naturally, being physically well also allows you to carry out duties that you otherwise would not be able to.

Keep moving: By maintaining a healthy lifestyle, you can participate in activities that need a specific level of physical fitness. For instance, mountain climbing is a rewarding activity that provides stunning scenery and a sense of accomplishment, yet there are certain people who cannot perform it due to physical limitations.

But for someone who doesn't regularly exercise, even going to the zoo with your family or taking your kids to the playground could be challenging. It is easier to keep up your level of activity as you become older if you are active.

Your health will improve: exercise has numerous advantageous consequences on your well-being. Regular exercise results in healthy bones and muscles. It improves overall health, respiratory health, and cardiovascular health. You can reduce your risk of developing some cancers, type 2 diabetes, and heart disease, and maintain a healthy weight by leading an active lifestyle.

In other words, maintaining fitness and good health depends on staying active. Encourage your family to be more active as you push yourself to meet daily or weekly physical activity goals. Set aside time to play sports outside with the entire family.

to go to the gym every day or to start a fit, healthy pastime like cycling or hiking. Increasing your exercise during National Physical Fitness and Sports Month is a great idea, but don't quit after the month is through. Make health and physical activity a regular part of your day!

Kids' physical activity: Children require varied amounts of exercise depending on their age. Between the ages of three and five, children must be active all day. Ages 6 through 17 must engage in 60 minutes of physical activity each day. even if it might feel like a lot. It's possible that children are exercising at the recommended levels already. You may also see ways to encourage youngsters to participate in enjoyable, age-appropriate, and varied activities.

Guidelines for Children between 3 and 5 years old

The adults who look after children should encourage active play. Recommendations for Children and Adolescents, Ages 6 to 17,

60 minutes or more of moderate to vigorous physical activity per day.

Exercises like walking, jogging, or other cardiovascular activities should take up the majority of the daily 60 minutes. There should be at least three days per week of vigorous-intensity exercise.

adding at least three days a week of pushups and other muscle-building workouts.

Exercises that strengthen the bones include jumping Additionally, kids can get the recommended 60 minutes of exercise each day with the help of school-based physical activity.

How can I know if my child is exercising aerobically at a high or low intensity?

On a scale of 0 to 10, where lying down is a 0 and the most passive condition is a 10, moderate activity is a 5 or 6. Children who modestly participate When engaged in rigorous exercise, people breathe deeper and their hearts beat faster than when they are at rest or seated motionless. Exercise at levels 7 or 8 is strenuous. Children who participate in intense activities breathe more deeply and have heart rates that are significantly higher than usual.

Another example is the moderately vigorous aerobic exercise that children engage in each morning as they walk to school with their friends. However, as they sprint or pursue after their opponents when playing tag at recess, children are probably engaging in vigorous-intensity activity.

There are some physical activities that are more suited for children than for teenagers. For instance, younger kids frequently practice gymnastics, play in a jungle gym, or climb trees to develop their muscles. It's common for kids to not need conventional muscle-building routines like weightlifting. Adolescent children are eligible to start formal weight-lifting exercises. These programs could be paired with the training they receive as a member of a sports team.

Older age routine:

One of the most important things you can do for your health as an older adult is to engage in regular physical activity. Many of the health problems associated with aging can be postponed or avoided by utilizing it. Additionally, it promotes muscle growth so you can keep working independently on daily duties.

Remember that exercise of any kind is better than none at all. Your health will benefit from physical activity more and more as you do it.

For people 65 and older, a minimum of 150 minutes per week (or 30 minutes per day, five days per week) of moderate-intensity activity is required, such as brisk walking. Or they need to exert themselves vigorously for 75 minutes each week by jogging, running, or climbing mountains.

Muscle-building workouts should be done at least two days per week.

in addition to exercises that improve balance, such as one-foot standing.

If chronic issues prevent you from following these recommendations, be as physically active as your abilities and conditions allow.

Chapter 2

A Fitter Way of Living,

As time goes on, many of us have made plans to enhance our physical and mental well-being. While having specific goals for your health and fitness is great, many people go above and above to attain these goals. They experiment with the newest trendy diet or exercise craze, which is frequently tiring. all of their physical and mental resources in the process.

Burnout, failure, or injury are common outcomes of this, as well as outright quitting or achieving these goals but being unable to maintain them. , So I advise you to attempt changing your way of life rather than setting totally unrealistic goals.

When you start to view health and fitness as a lifelong decision rather than a fleeting interest or a 30-day goal, you develop behaviors that will improve many aspects of your life.

You may be more creative and have more self-control, flexibility, and balance if you have a healthy lifestyle. By doing this, you'll not only feel and look better, but you'll be able to portray a better version of yourself to the people who matter most in your life.

THESE RULES GO BEYOND AESTHETICS:
Health and fitness matter more than just how you look, what you eat, or how much weight you can lift at the gym. They are

connected to your mental health as well as your ability to focus at work, move about, and generally feel well.

Your attitude and physical skills are higher when you are physically well. Trekking, paddleboarding, or walking your dog are all options. If you are unable to engage in these activities, it may have a negative influence on your experiences and quality of life.

Be an example for others to follow.
By making the decision to live a healthy lifestyle, you not only benefit yourself but everyone else as well. Your friends, family, and children are affected by the healthy decisions you make, and they frequently feel inspired to make changes in their own lives as a result.

The outcomes of this are better relationships, a lower risk of illness, and a generally healthier and happier planet. The simple act of making better choices could benefit everyone in your surrounding area. Start the transformation on your own.

YOU LEARN EXACT BEHAVIORAL CHANGES

I've learned that "diets" and "workout challenges" only last so long. It is not practicable to always travel at 100 mph. We are all human. Life happens, conflicts arise and disappear, and plans occasionally get derailed.

When we choose to live a healthy lifestyle, we learn to ADAPT. You learn to enjoy life when you are on vacation and away from your kitchen and gym because you have developed the habits and skills to lead a healthy lifestyle wherever you are. If you routinely exercise moderation and balance, you may treat yourself without going overboard. If you don't have access to a gym for one week, you get into the habit of bringing your resistance bands with you when you travel, creating a bodyweight circuit, or exercising on the nearby stairs and benches. You learn to adjust when your pattern is disturbed rather than self-destruct.

Yes, people can attain results by following strict workout routines or extreme diets. However, very few people actually follow through on these plans. These jobs are typically completed fast and have strict success and failure criteria, neither of which are good for your mental or emotional health. If you set unrealistic goals, you are more likely to suffer failure. When the expectations are lower, you are more likely to stick with it and enjoy your journey. You don't hold yourself to this standard of perfection. If you eat something "bad" or skip a workout, you wake up the next day and go right back on track since it has become a habit. This method is easier to implement and yields results that are more reliable over time.

Make health and fitness a habit of life right immediately with the advice provided below:

1. Select an activity that you enjoy: This is essential if you want to keep your exercise regimen consistent. If you frequently engage in uncomfortable physical activity that depletes both your physical and emotional energy, it will only last so long. It's crucial to choose routines that you enjoy and can stick with over the long term, even if they aren't the most demanding. Regular low-intensity exercise is always preferable to sporadic high-intensity 5exercise in terms of effectiveness.

2. As you attempt to accomplish your physical objectives, be patient:

Remember that development takes time. Be kind to yourself. Nothing worth having is easy. Gain the ability to accept the journey, the people you encounter, and the process.

3. Continue to consume the items you like: You should always consume the foods you prefer, in my opinion. Discover a more wholesome way to make your favorite recipes. If pizza is one of your favorite foods, keep eating it. As a result, you will feel starved. Utilize creative thinking and fresh ingredients to make your own healthy version.

4. NEVER compete with someone: This is where your life and your adventure begin. As no two people are alike, you shouldn't ever compare yourself to others. As long as you get up every day and try to get better, you are on the right track.

5. Attempt novel stuff:

Step outside of your comfort zone. Visit different restaurants and enroll with a friend in an exercise class. Doing your grocery shopping in accordance with what's in season is an easy way to start experimenting with new dishes and exposing yourself to a wide variety of fruits and vegetables. Try meal planning if you haven't already! It will keep things interesting and encourage and motivate you to adopt this style of living. So get outside your comfort zone and experiment.

One of the most crucial things you can do to maintain optimum health is to include exercise in your daily routine. People who are at a healthy weight and are physically active live, on average, seven years longer than those who are obese and don't exercise. Being active helps to prevent or delay chronic diseases and disorders associated with aging. As a result, active people maintain their independence and quality of life for longer.

Fitness is a quality or state of being in a physically healthy and fit state. The word "fitness" increased by a factor of 10 in Western slang. The ability of a human or a machine to perform a certain task or, more broadly, the ability of a person to adapt to a variety of settings is the current definition of fitness. The relationship between physical attractiveness and human fitness has driven the global fitness and fitness equipment industries. Fitness is defined as having a significant anaerobic or aerobic capacity (i.e., strength or endurance) for a certain function. A well-rounded fitness program, such as one that focuses exclusively on cardio/respiratory exercise or weight training, enhances a person's fitness in all areas as opposed to just one.

Many sources stress the significance of mental, social, and emotional health as components of general fitness. A full fitness plan intended for a given person typically stresses one or more special abilities, as well as age- or health-related criteria like bone health. This is sometimes depicted in textbooks as a triangle with three points, one for each of the three types of health: physical, emotional, and mental. Maintaining a healthy weight has been shown to aid in disease prevention and hasten the recovery time following an injury or illness. Fitness has been shown to have positive effects on both physical and mental health, addressing anxiety and depression in addition to the benefits of physical health. Given that it has the potential to both prevent and treat a wide range of other chronic health issues brought on by unhealthy lifestyles or aging, physical activity has long been regarded as one of the most popular and helpful self-care practices. Exercise can help some individuals sleep better and may even help some people with their mood issues by raising their sleep pressure.

Recent research has demonstrated that many of the benefits of exercise are mediated by the skeletal muscle's role as an endocrine organ. To put it another way, myokines are a group of chemicals that are released when muscles contract. These myokines can promote the growth of new tissue and tissue healing in addition to having a variety of anti-inflammatory actions.

Chapter 3

macros and tracker

The nutrients known as macronutrients—abbreviated "macros"—are those that your body needs to carry out routine actions and processes. The three basic macronutrients are protein, fat, and carbohydrates, and each one serves a certain purpose in your body. The advantages of eating the proper ratio of protein, fats, and carbohydrates are many and include: "Everything the body does, from exercise to breathing, requires carbohydrates; Fats make up the body's cells, help us absorb vitamins, play a role in heart health, and help us feel full longer; while protein helps maintain muscle and bone health, helps control diabetes, and repairs cells."

There is no recommended daily intake for macronutrients, and your requirements will change based on your sex, height, weight, degree of exercise, and personal goals. Women are advised to get between 45 and 65 percent of their calories from carbohydrates, 20 to 35 percent from fats, and 10 to 35 percent from protein, according to the United States Department of Agriculture.

These general guidelines might help you decide how much of your meal to devote to each macronutrient. But some people, such as those trying to achieve a health or performance objective or people with specific medical issues, may prefer to estimate the precise number of macronutrients they require and pay greater attention to their consumption (more on the reasons why in a moment).

Make accurate macro calculations: To calculate the correct quantity of each macronutrient you need, you must first calculate how many calories you burn each day.

Additionally, you need to know how many calories each gram of each macronutrient contains: 1 gram of fat contains 9 calories, 1 gram of protein contains 4 calories, and 1 gram of carbs includes 4 calories. Next, take out a notebook and utilize the following two basic formulas:

Daily Calories Per Macro: total daily calories multiplied by the number of calories from a particular macronutrient each day.

Daily grams per macro: daily calories of the macronutrient. Calories per gram of the macronutrient

For illustration, a person who consumes 2,000 calories daily would calculate their macros as follows:

Carbohydrates
- 1000 such calories are equal to 2000 total calories times 50 of a calorie's worth of carbohydrates.
- 1000 calories from carbohydrates are provided by 250 grams of carbohydrates per day or 4 calories from each gram of carbohydrates.
- 600 calories are obtained by multiplying 2000 total calories by the 30 that come from fat.
- 67 grams of fat per day, or 9 calories per gram of fat, from 600 calories of fat.

Protein:

- o   400 such calories are obtained by multiplying 2000 total calories by 20 grams of protein per calorie.
- o   400 calories of protein, or 4 calories per gram, provide 100 grams of protein each day.

Again, these recommendations for protein, fat, and carbohydrate intake are merely guidelines; individual calorie and macronutrient needs may differ. For instance, compared to someone who prefers to unwind on the couch most days, someone who runs every morning undoubtedly needs to eat more carbohydrates.

Maintaining Macros

By tracking your macros, you may be able to reduce your weight, improve the quality of your diet, and reach specific health-related goals. It involves determining your nutrient needs and monitoring your intake with a food journal or an app.

If you frequent a gym or keep up with the health scene, you've probably heard of "counting macros."

You can accomplish a number of health goals by counting macronutrients (macros), which is typically done by people who want to gain muscle or reduce weight.

It's important to monitor your calorie intake and the types of foods you eat in order to reach certain macronutrient and calorie goals.

Even though counting macros is quite simple, it can be challenging if you're just getting started.

Let me outline the benefits of macro counting and walk you through the process in detail.

Although it takes some effort to learn how to measure macronutrients, anyone may use the method.

To determine your total calorie needs, you must calculate your non-resting energy expenditure (NREE) and resting energy expenditure (REE).

Calories expended when exercising and digesting food are referred to as NREE, whilst calories burned while at rest are referred to as REE.

Adding REE and NREE results in total daily energy expenditure (TDEE) often referred to as daily caloric expenditure (DCE).

Either a straightforward online calculator or the Mifflin-St. To determine your overall calorie needs, use the Jeor equation:

For males, calories per day equal 10 times their weight in kilograms, 6.25 times their height in centimeters, five times their age in years, and five for females.

After that, the result is multiplied by an activity factor, which is a number that represents different levels of activity.

- 1.2 times sedentary (little exercise)
- Less than three days per week of light exercise: x 1.375
- An average of 1.55 days per week are spent engaging in moderate activity.
- Very active (daily, hard exercise): x 1.725
- Extra-active: x 1.9 (engaged in strenuous activities twice daily or more)

- o The final result is supplied, which is your TDEE.
- o Calories can be added to or subtracted from your overall expenditure to achieve a variety of goals.

In other words, if you want to lose weight, you should consume fewer calories than you burn off, and if you want to gain muscle, you should consume more calories.

The Options for Macros Monitoring

Although not everyone needs to, some people might find it handy to keep track of their macros. Additionally, "calculating your macros allows you to know what to shoot for - what your objective is, regardless of the motivation." Additionally, "knowing how many messages and strategies are available may help someone set goals because there are so many of them."

Similarly, people with chronic renal disease frequently need to restrict their protein intake to better manage their illness, and monitoring their macronutrients can help them make sure they don't consume more than is advised. People with certain medical disorders, such as type I diabetes, may refer to their macronutrient consumption to ensure they match the grams of carbohydrates they ingest at meals to an insulin dosage.

To ensure that their body stays in ketosis, which occurs when the body burns fat instead of glucose stored in the body, someone who follows the ketogenic diet, which calls for getting 75% of their calories from fat, 20% from protein, and 5% from carbohydrates, may also want to monitor their macronutrients, especially their carb and fat intake.

People who want to lose weight, gain muscle mass, or accomplish a performance goal might also choose to calculate and track their macros,

An endurance athlete training for an Ironman event may benefit from monitoring their carb intake to ensure they are providing their body with enough of the energy source it needs to function at such a high intensity.

The Problems with Calculating Using Macros

Caution should be exercised when using your calculated macros to guide your meal decisions: "Just because you consume 'x quantity' of macros does not guarantee that they are of high quality. One might have a diet rich in processed foods and still meet macronutrient goals if they are only concerned with the distribution of macronutrients in their diet. Yes, consuming protein bars and high-fat, low-carb sweets may help you reach your daily recommended macronutrient intake, but they may also be poor in fiber and other important micronutrients.

A lot of mental work is required to maintain macro objectives, and for some people, this focus on numbers can result in an unhealthy relationship with food. "I highly advise people to redirect their focus, time, and energy to anything else.

I say that adding macro counting to what we already have on our plates is needless! [Counting your macros] needs a lot of concentration and willpower, so avoid doing it unless you really must.

Do You Need to Calculate Your Macros Now?

Given the commitment and work required to meet your protein, fat, and carbohydrate targets, as well as the chance that doing so can have a negative effect on your health —

"Tracing macros is not necessary for good eating. Focus on the quality of your meals and what food combinations make you feel physically and emotionally full rather than counting grams.

And if you do choose to calculate your macros after speaking with a qualified nutritionist, I strongly advise you not to let those figures define you.

In addition, remember that you shouldn't let it turn into an obsession that consumes valuable brain space that you could use for a variety of other productive activities in your life. "Keep an eye on your macros to the extent that it promotes the creation of a consistent eating schedule and eating habits for you.

Chapter 4

Cardiovascular Benefits

There are many different cardiovascular workouts, but the most important factors for achieving your fitness goals are consistency, length, and intensity. Read on to learn more about this form of exercise, its benefits, and how to design a safe and effective cardiovascular program.

Cardio, also known as aerobic exercise, is any rhythmic exercise that drives your heart rate into the optimal heart rate range. It is in this heart rate range that you burn the most calories and fat.

Even ordinary domestic duties like sweeping and cleaning can count as heart exercise. The most common cardio exercises include swimming, cycling, and walking.

Numerous factors may influence an individual's cardiac capacity or aptitude. Cardio varies from other forms of exercise, such as weight training, in part because it depends on your body's ability to utilize oxygen during the workout.

The ability to exercise your heart can be affected by heredity by 20% to 40%, according to a study by the American Heart Association.1 Additionally, the cardiac capacity of both sexes tends to decline with age and is typically 25% lower in females than in males.

However, it is helpful to be aware that a number of factors might affect how (and how well) your body responds to cardiac activity.

This is not to imply that you can't enhance your cardiovascular health regardless of your genes, sex, or age.

Benefits of Cardio

Cardio exercise helps you burn fat and calories, which makes it easier to lose weight. Cardio exercise has many advantages for your physical and mental health that few quick-time hobbies can match. especially if the activity is moderate to intense in nature, enhances the quality of sleep by increasing lung capacity, You can increase the amount of air that your lungs can hold.

The ability of your body to become aroused is increased, your perception of your body is improved, and it may even help alleviate sexual dysfunction brought on by medicine. Your bone density rises as you take part in weight-bearing aerobic exercises like hiking or stair climbing. Encourages positive emotions and may even be able to relieve depression and anxiety6 Boosts self-confidence in terms of how you feel and seem. Reduces stress in part by improving your capacity for constructive problem-solving. lowers the risk of heart attack, diabetes, high blood pressure, high cholesterol, and a number of cancers7

sets a good example for everyone around you, encouraging them to get some exercise. strengthens the heart, requiring less work from the organ to pump blood.

How to Choose a Cardio Exercise

The first step in choosing the best cardio workout for you is determining the types of activities you enjoy. Take into account what you would feel comfortable incorporating into your life and what suits your personality. This is important since you won't be as likely to stick with the exercise routine over time if you don't enjoy it.

If you like to work out at the gym, there are several options available, including treadmills, elliptical trainers, climbers, stationary cycles, and more. There are several delightful outdoor activities, including cycling, walking, and running.

You can do aerobic exercises at home like burpees, jumping jacks, running while stationary, and jumping rope. Another option is to get your own elliptical or treadmill machine. You can also think about using: workout DVDs. App to help you get in shape

Don't be afraid to try anything and, if it doesn't work, move on to something else because this process might be hit or miss. For example, exercise sandbags may provide a whole-body workout with just one piece of equipment. If you don't know what you enjoy, try a variety of activities to find out which one or the ones you like most.

Newcomer's Exercises

If you've never exercised before, there are a few beginner routines that might help you get started.

Cardio for Complete Newbies: With this application, you can use whatever machine or exercise you like.

Elliptical exercise for beginners: Because it has a gentle impact and is therefore better for your joints, the elliptical machine is great for building strength.

Try this 20-minute indoor cycling routine if you want a low-impact workout for beginners.

You should be at Level 5 or 6 on a scale of zero to 10, where sitting is zero and the utmost amount of effort that can be put out is 10. Another option is to start with roughly 10 to 20 minutes of brisk, moderate-intensity walking.

How long should an aerobic workout last?

Health regulators recommend that most adults perform 150 minutes of cardiovascular activity each week.8 The benefit of cardio is that you don't have to work out for an hour to see results.

Decide how much work you must accomplish each week and break it up in a way that makes sense to you. Even 10-minute sessions count toward your weekly requirements for cardiac activity.

If you're just getting started, breaking up your sessions into 10- to 15-minute chunks could feel less frightening. As the exercise becomes easier, increase the time allotted for each session by five minutes, eventually moving up to sessions lasting 30 to 60 minutes.

frequency of cardio workouts

Your level of fitness, schedule, and goals are just a few of the factors that determine how often you should undertake aerobic workouts.

Cardio three to four times a week is probably enough if you have been working out consistently for years, are used to working out for 60 minutes at a time, and prioritize muscle growth over fat burning. If you are new to exercise, want to be healthy, don't have a lot of free time, and are concerned about losing weight, a small amount of exercise each day can be beneficial.

When talking about frequency, it's important to consider both frequency and intensity. Cardio exercises that are light to moderate in intensity can frequently be done every day, whereas high-intensity exercise requires more days off between workouts. Combining the two helps to prevent burnout and promotes the use of different energy systems.

Cardio Frequency Guidelines

The frequency of your workouts will depend on your level of fitness and availability. The basic guidelines are:

For general health, try 30 minutes of moderately intense exercise five days a week, or 20 minutes of intense cardio three days a week.

To meet your goals for weight loss and/or to avoid gaining weight, you may need to perform more than 300 minutes of moderate-intensity exercise per week.

To maintain a healthy body weight, you need between 150 and 300 minutes of moderate-intensity exercise per week.

Keep it moderate (three to six days a week, depending on your level of fitness), vary your effort, and don't forget to take rest days when necessary because there is a point of diminishing returns when performing too much cardio.

When Reality Snatches You

The transition to more consistent exercise may take a few weeks if you're still working on increasing your endurance and conditioning. What happens if you are unable to follow the rules?

Despite any obstacles, such as a busy schedule, try your best to exercise as often as you can. To make the most of the time you do have, try using circuit training activities that are shorter but more intense.

Low-impact cardio exercise that uses your own body weight as resistance for 10 minutes without the usage of any extra equipment

Six different exercise options are provided in Burn 10 Minutes to Burn 100 Calories to keep things interesting.

You may need to change your lifestyle if you are unable to put forth the necessary effort to achieve your goals. If that doesn't work, change your objective to match where you are in your workout or weight loss experience. Keep in mind that you may struggle to lose weight if you can't follow the instructions due to a busy schedule.

Exercise Hardness for Heart

Your workout will be greatly influenced by how hard you work because of: Your workout will be greatly influenced by how hard you work because:

Calorie burn: There is a direct relationship between intensity and the number of calories you burn.

Monitoring is simple: Using a heart rate monitor or the perceived exertion scale, you may easily monitor the intensity of your workout.

time reduction Increase your effort to burn more calories when time is of the essence.

Variation: You don't have to find a new exercise to do to change the intensity of your workout.

By using adjustable kettlebells, you may combine strength training with cardio while adjusting the level of difficulty.

You can choose to focus on one of three different degrees of intensity throughout your workouts, or you can mix all three levels into one session, depending on your fitness level and goals:

If you want to exert more effort for shorter periods of time, try beginning interval training. High-Intensity Cardio: This type of exercise requires your heart rate to be between 70% and 85% of its maximum (MHR), or a 7 or 8 on the scale of perceived effort.

It's difficult for you to talk for very long at this level since you're out of breath..

Cardio with a Moderate Intensity: The U.S. Department of Health and Human Services frequently suggests this degree of intensity in its Physical Activity Guidelines. Usually, when working out, you want to aim for this level.

Cardio with a Moderate Intensity: Between 50% and 70% of your MHR (levels 5 to 6 on the scale of perceived exertion) is considered moderate intensity.

Low-Intensity Cardio: When you warm up or squeeze in other workouts during the day, like strolling, you should work at this level. This type of activity is rated as being between levels 3 and 4 on the scale of perceived effort, or below 50% of your MHR.

Exercise to Lose Weight:
Actual exercise requirements for weight loss are frequently higher; you may need 300 minutes of exercise per week or more if you want to lose more than 5% of your body weight. According to the Physical Activity Guidelines for Americans, the majority of adults should exercise for 150 minutes each week at a moderate level.

These guidelines define moderate-intensity exercise as any activity that increases heart rate, but they also opine that adding HIIT frequently produces better results for people who are overweight or obese.

Combining weight training with your regular exercise regimen may also be beneficial since it builds lean muscle, which uses more energy than fat10 and raises calorie expenditure both at rest and during exercise.

The Dietary Guidelines for Americans recommend avoiding added sugar, saturated fat, salt, and alcohol while consuming adequate fruits, vegetables, grains, low-fat dairy, lean meats, and healthy oils.11 You may expedite weight loss by adding exercise to a balanced diet.

It gets easier as you practice more, so keep your cardio activities basic at all times. Start small and establish a daily goal to do something, even if it's only a little stroll. Schedule it in your calendar and try to do it at the same time each day.

Chapter 5

The Benefits of Rest and Recuperation

If you regularly work out and are wondering why you aren't getting the results you want in terms of performance, strength improvements, or weight reduction, it may be because your schedule doesn't allow enough time for rest and recovery.

Not just "a nice break from your program," rest and recovery are an essential part of your planned and deliberate training regimen.

There are two elements

Strength training in particular tears tiny rips in the muscles that your body needs to mend and adapt, resulting in you becoming slightly stronger than before as a result of the adaptation, enabling you to handle more load in the future. However, depending on the activities you engage in, this process might take anywhere from 48 to 72 hours.

Thus, the goal of resting is to free you up to exercise more, benefit more from your routines, and ultimately achieve higher results.

Rest also gives you a chance to replenish your glycogen stores, which your muscles and liver use during activity as a temporary energy source.

This is depleted during exercise, especially cardiac exercise. For these reserves to replenish and be ready for your next training session, it requires 48 hours and an adequate diet. The objective is to improve your ability to put up greater effort during exercises and your long-term training results.

Second, not getting enough rest and sleep causes your hormones to go out of balance. Training is a "stressor," designed to put your muscles under pressure and force them to respond by producing more growth hormone, which promotes development. However, your body is unable to distinguish between everyday stressors and those associated with training, which causes your levels of naturally occurring cortisol to rise.

Lack of "life stress management," namely not getting enough sleep, results in poor insulin sensitivity, lower levels of the hormone connected to appetite suppression (leptin), and increased levels of the hormone linked to hunger (ghrelin). This basically means that no matter how hard you work, you will probably still have body fat, and that you won't respond to training as you should (which is the opposite of what you want).

You should be able to achieve incredible consistency in your training while still being in a state that encourages prolonged, positive adaptation by reducing life pressures and increasing your training load. Getting enough rest, recovering, and eating healthily to complement your training are the best ways to achieve this.

How can you determine if you are exercising too much or not enough?

The fact that you are maintaining body fat despite your exercise and that your performance is not improving are the two most obvious signs that you are not giving yourself enough time for rest and recovery. However, there are additional, important warning signs to look out for.

- You can feel drowsy all day long from poor-quality, fragmented sleep, but be wide awake and unable to fall asleep at night. There may be additional symptoms, such as nighttime sweats.
- Poor results in competitions or while training - Despite your best efforts, you are unable to develop the necessary intensity, power, and performance. A lot of work is perceived throughout training. Your body hurts, and over time you're beginning to injure yourself.
- Overtraining and an imbalance in your training program are clearly indicated by muscular soreness after exercise and the onset of overuse injuries. When your muscles and tendons are unable to adapt to the microtrauma of training and the degree of breakdown is greater than the degree of healing, a severe stop to your training may be necessary due to an injury you may not be able to manage.
- Your immune system is weak (as a result of overexertion and high cortisone levels) if you get sick more frequently and recover from diseases more slowly. Other signs could be a change in appetite (either more or decreased satiety) or more serious blood markers including low vitamin D, low iron, and high levels of creatine kinase (a marker for muscle breakdown).
- Simply said, your thinking might not feel right. When you no longer want to train, feel unfulfilled by training or making progress toward your goals, or experience

feelings of despair or melancholy, your mind is trying to alert you that you are burnt out and need to obtain enough rest and recovery.

What makes a rehabilitation program effective?

Just like effective training, excellent recovery should be incorporated into your workout program. Schedule your key training sessions first so that you can give them everything you have. This will allow you to organize your relaxation and recovery afterward.

The main exercise type is strength training. two to three times a week. You exert most of your work here in order to progressively build up your strength and perform better. These exercises are specifically created to improve your strength in both your weak regions and areas where performance is required.

To monitor your improvement and adaptation throughout the course of several sessions, it is imperative that you gradually increase the intensity of your training. The keys to success are consistency, method, steady overload, and improvement. It is expected that you will feel fatigued after these sessions because this is where the job is done.

The three sessions that make up a week may be scheduled on Monday, Wednesday, or Friday, or for Tuesday, Thursday, and Saturday.

It is important to give the body ample time to heal so that growth and repair can occur.

 2-3 times a week, primary cardiovascular and primary strength training should take place on the same day.

If you are preparing for a cardio event like a triathlon, a marathon run, or a sport like netball or football, your primary cardio training days should be on your strength training days.

Strength training should preferably be spread out over a period of 48 hours even though this sort of cardiac activity recovers in about 3–4 hours. Strength training and cardio should therefore be combined for the best results and a day of rest the following day.

To be effective, this session must be difficult, much like strength training. In order to improve performance, this does not suggest a leisurely run but rather sprint training, speed work, or possibly interval training. You need to put in more effort than usual if you want to advance and adapt; otherwise, your outcomes will stay the same.

The optimal workouts for you to achieve your goals without pushing yourself too hard and running the risk of injury will be determined by a competent coach.

However, both of these workouts require a recovery period in order for your body to recuperate and for you to exercise again at your best.

The day following your harder training days is your "post-exercise rest day."

These days are intended to stimulate blood circulation and allow the body to recuperate. This will aid in the breakdown of the exercise metabolite creatine kinase.k

On these days, exercise should Be performed at a conversational speed Last no longer than an hour (ideally under 40 minutes).

These are the ideal days to take your significant other for a stroll or a leisurely ride. Avoid going overboard on these days as doing so will prevent you from recovering and giving your best effort on your harder training days.

• Additional light training days: If you work out twice weekly, choose the day after your recuperation day OR the day before your first heavier training day of the week.

Although the emphasis is on honing your sport's technical elements, talents, and techniques, these are still lighter sessions. Use these days to increase your technical knowledge, saving your assigned training days for performance enhancement.

Additional recovery-related support measures is to Get enough rest: 7 hours every night on average. This is the most important restorative exercise you can do. This is the best method to lessen "non-training stress" and lower cortisol levels. The majority of healing takes place during this time, thus your performance will decrease if your sleep is interrupted.

You may need to forego other social engagements or say NO to unneeded commitments in order to ensure that you get enough, high-quality sleep as part of your whole training routine.

According to research, an athlete's objective is to reduce non-training stressors in order to maximize adaptation to each applied unit of training stress. An athlete frequently makes an effort to simplify their lives, cut back on or completely avoid "normal" work schedules, and give sleep a priority.

Nutritious meals that your body can use as fuel while exercising and to grow

Food (energy) should be your fuel while exercising. Your performance declines and your results are impaired when you undereat while exercising.

Your body's capacity for healing and growth will be hampered if you skip eating before working out. Consuming some carbs prior to exercise, high-quality protein, and water for hydration are all required for the optimal effects of exercise.

When you eat high-quality protein within 30 minutes of working out and a complete meal with protein, unrefined carbohydrates from fruits and vegetables, and high-quality fats within two hours of working out, you have the best chance of getting the most out of your workout and maximizing your gains.

Rest and recovery are essential parts of any fitness plan, especially for professional athletes.

The importance of exercise training for raising performance is recognized by athletes. Rest and recuperation, however, are equally essential parts of an exercise program since they offer the body time in between workouts to strengthen and restore itself. It also enables the athlete to recover mentally and physically.

Exercise puts the body under stress, giving it time to repair damaged body tissue and refill muscle glycogen (energy stores).

Two types of recovery can be distinguished:
Immediate or short-term recovery occurs most frequently just after an exercise session or other activity. Short-term healing includes low-intensity exercise after working out and throughout the cool-down time.

Long-term recovery is the phrase used to describe periods of rest that are part of a seasonal training schedule and may last for several days or weeks within an annual sporting schedule.

Sleep is yet another essential aspect of rest and recovery when it comes to sports performance. In addition to increasing cortisol levels (a stress hormone) and decreasing human growth hormone, which is essential in tissue regeneration, lack of sleep puts athletes in danger of losing aerobic endurance.

If you are a high-level athlete or have a family member who plays a sport that demands a higher level of fitness, it is recommended that you keep track of your workouts using a training log. You can use a training log to keep note of how your body responds to exercise; this will allow you to determine your recovery requirements and whether your training regimen needs to be adjusted.

Chapter 6

Important Supplements for Rest and Recovery

Some supplements have been scientifically proven to enhance post-workout recovery and repair, but they cannot take the place of refueling with food, hydration, and relaxation after strenuous activity. What you should know about vitamins for recovery is provided here.

Intense stretching and relaxing activities break down muscle cells and microscopic breaks in muscle fibers, increasing blood flow to the damaged muscle and causing inflammation (which can be beneficial for healing). There may also be some muscle discomfort. A workout's recovery is just as crucial as the exertion itself.

With appropriate recovery, the short-term inflammation goes down, the muscle is repaired (and can regenerate even stronger), and the discomfort goes down, allowing you to get back to high-intensity exercise more quickly.

Early exercise, however, can result in muscular damage, including inflammation, delayed onset muscle soreness, increased feelings of weariness, and the disruption and breakdown of proteins in muscle fibers and connective tissues, if the right precautions aren't taken to give your body time to recuperate.

How do vitamins help with muscle recovery?

Some supplements may provide you a much-needed healing boost, while it's not a good idea to rely on them as your main means of recovery.

- o   promoting muscle synthesis (growth)
- o   reducing muscular pain
- o   increased blood flow
- o   eliminating inflammation
- o   lowering the sense of tiredness

Let's examine the science supporting these five supplements for muscle restoration.

Being the most abundant protein in the body and an essential component of connective tissues including tendons, ligaments, and cartilage, collagen supplements may be able to relieve joint pain.

In comparison to other protein supplements like whey, collagen is higher in the amino acids glycine, proline, and hydroxyproline — all of which are necessary for synthesizing collagen in the body. Collagen supplements are typically sold as powders and may be labeled as "collagen," "hydrolyzed collagen," "collagen hydrolysate," or "collagen peptides."

Collagen supplements aid in the healing process for patients and athletes who have joint pain by:

An athlete can experience less joint pain in as short as 12 weeks.

Extending the amount of time spent exercising pain-free

improved knee joint extension

The recommended dosage for collagen supplements ranges from 5 to 15 g per day, and they can be taken at any time of the day, even before or after exercise.

There are two main cherry types: sweet and tart. Sweet cherries are typically taken fresh; sour cherries are sometimes turned into juice or are dried, powdered, and capsuled as supplements.

According to numerous studies, taking tart cherry supplements can speed up recovery by lowering inflammation and muscular discomfort, preserving strength, boosting the body's antioxidant defenses, and reducing soreness and pain in the muscles. Tart cherries are full of antioxidants that help prevent muscle injury and recuperation by acting as a vasodilator, which increases blood flow and provides the damaged muscles with the oxygen and nutrients they need to heal.

For instance, a 2016 study looked at how elite male athletes responded to 30 mL of tart cherry concentrate in water five days before and three days after a lengthy, repeated sprint and agility training session. The findings showed that individuals taking the tart cherry supplement recovered more quickly than the group receiving a placebo, with lower rates of muscular soreness and a decreased inflammatory response.

The ideal dosage depends on the type of supplement (juice, concentrate, or supplements), the extent and duration of the workout, and the form used. To aid in recuperation, tart cherries can be consumed as juice, concentrate, or supplements days before, the day of, and days after a physically demanding event.

Malate of citrulline:

Citrulline is actually converted to arginine in the body, which may help with recuperation. Citrulline and malate combine to generate citrulline malate, which is an important component of energy synthesis.

by widening the blood arteries to boost circulation

eliminating ammonium from your system (which may help to reduce muscle fatigue)

One study of 41 men found that a single supplement dose of citrulline malate was associated with a 53% increase in barbell bench press repetitions and lower levels of fatigue, while a smaller study of 15 resistance-trained women found that short-term citrulline malate supplementation improved perceived exertion during both a bench press and lower body exercise.

What you should know before taking supplements: Studies show that an effective dose of citrulline malate may vary from 8 to 12 g. For trained athletes—not those who only occasionally engage in mild or moderate exercise—citrulline malate can have an impact on both performance and recuperation.

Branch chain amino acid (BCAA) supplements: Valine, leucine, and isoleucine are the three necessary amino acids that must be received through diet as the body is unable to produce them on its own. Because amino acids are the building blocks of protein, BCAA supplements can encourage the synthesis of muscular protein, which leads to muscle growth and strength.

BCAA supplements, which are often available as a powder and coupled with a liquid like water, have been used by the athletic community for decades. The supplement may provide benefits, but such benefits are subject to some restrictions.

A 2017 evaluation of 11 clinical research indicated that the biggest recovery effects were observed when a high daily dose of BCAAs was ingested for at least 10 days. This means that supplementing with BCAAs isn't a quick fix: you can't own a BCAA shake after a strenuous workout and expect it to work.

The overall protein concentration of these supplements typically tends to be larger (20-25g per serving) than that of a standalone BCAA supplement. Some whey, soy, or other plant-based protein powders may contain BCAA. You can consume BCAA supplements before and/or after working out. Despite more studies being done on men than on women, BCAAs may speed up recovery by reducing muscle pain and protein synthesis.

The primary active component of turmeric, curcumin, which is also sold as a supplement, serves as an antioxidant and lowers inflammation in the body.

A 2020 review published in Nutrients that looked at data from 11 studies with a total of 237 participants found that supplementing with 150–1,500 mg of curcumin daily reduced perceived muscle pain, decreased creatine kinase levels (a blood enzyme that indicates muscle damage), and improved muscle performance. By preventing the action of pro-inflammatory chemicals, curcumin also aids in the reduction of post-workout inflammation.

Before taking supplements, you should be aware that while curcumin is naturally found in turmeric, you'll need considerably greater doses to experience the spice's healing effects. You can use supplements containing curcumin before, during, or after working exercise.

Fish oil supplements contain omega-3 fatty acids EPA and DHA, which are known for being anti-inflammatory and heart-healthy.

While the optimal dosage to accomplish this advantage is still unknown, one seven-week clinical investigation revealed that supplementing with 6g daily showed the most benefit when compared to 2g or 4g doses, while other studies reported that 1g to 2g daily doses produced appreciable improvements. By easing muscular aches and enhancing measurements like range of motion and maximum voluntary contraction, fish oil supplements may aid in recuperation.

There is presently inadequate research to show whether this is a successful technique to enhance recovery for females. Studies have mostly focused on the benefits of this supplement in male athletes [18–20]. Supplemental fish oil may reduce muscular pain and increase the range of motion after exercise.

choose the best recovery aid available
A diet gap should be filled with supplements as well. You might want to think about taking a collagen supplement if your objective is to relieve joint pain following exercise. If reducing post-exercise inflammation is your goal, curcumin or tart cherry juice would be a better option. Add-ons are not a focused strategy for nutrition or muscle repair.

A healthy post-workout recovery is essential for building and maintaining muscle mass and preventing injury. Some supplements can speed up blood flow, lessen fatigue, and reduce inflammation, which can all help the body's healing processes

There is proof that supplements including fish oil, collagen, tart cherry juice, citrulline malate, BCAAs, and tart cherry juice can help active persons recuperate from workouts.

When selecting supplements to consume, take into account your goals and present diet.

If you are unsure of where to start, seek specialist, personalized counsel.

Creatine kinase, testosterone, cortisol, vitamin D, the liver enzymes ALT and AST, and hsCRP are among the biomarkers associated with recovery that are measured by The Ultimate and Immunity Plan, two of InsideTracker's blood plans. Most of these biomarkers aren't present in routine blood tests conducted at your doctor's office.

In addition to providing the raw data for these indicators, InsideTracker also informs you of their optimization status and offers ideas to enhance underperforming biomarkers based on scientific research. You might even come across suggestions for the vitamins on this list, along with suggested dosages!

To view InsideTracker plans, You have the option to select the Injury prevention/recovery target in both the Ultimate and Immunity Plans, which gives precedence to recommendations that help your body recover from workouts and reduce your risk of injury from subsequent exercises.

Chapter 7

How to control your sweet taste

It turns out that cravings for sugar are commonly brought on by prolonged training. Consequently, it is a habit. You have an action, a trigger, and a benefit.

Dopamine is the hormone that makes us feel happy after eating our favorite dessert, while insulin controls how much sugar is in our blood. The primitive brain regions that make up our reward system experience an increase in insulin when we consume sugar. Dopamine is released more frequently as a result, making us feel happier. Finishing supper may serve as the stimulus, consuming sweets may serve as the action, and feeling good may serve as the reward.

Finding a healthy substitute habit will help you break the habit of overindulging in sweets after meals and "reprogram your brain." Because your brain genuinely misses a rewarding habit when you stop doing it, cravings are likely to become stronger and difficult to control. Instead of dessert, treat yourself to something else: This might be talking on the phone with a friend, watching your favorite program, or taking a relaxing bath.

Some studies suggest that the absence of some beneficial bacteria, such as Lactobacillus johnsonii, can also cause cravings, possibly through the reduction of GABA production. Pathogenic gut bacteria use sugar as one of their nutritional sources, so the craving is really the bacteria signaling it wants its food to multiply.

Poor gut health, gut inflammation, and other G.I. tract problems are other possible reasons for sugar cravings. Improve the health of your gut flora to satisfy sugar cravings; if that doesn't work, see a doctor.

You may alter a few aspects of your lifestyle, including how you eat, to naturally improve the health of your gut microbiota. The best ways to do this are to consume lots of high-fiber meals, eat more probiotic foods (think: fermented foods), and consume foods that will help to reduce inflammation.

Whole grains, fruits, and vegetables are examples of foods high in fiber that can help reduce the absorption of sugar into the circulation and avoid blood sugar increases. Additionally, protein-rich meals like lean meats, beans, and lentils can help control blood sugar by encouraging feelings of fullness and slowing down digestion.

If you've ever wondered why you feel the need to indulge in ice cream after a difficult day, it may have something to do with your serotonin levels. It makes perfect sense that our systems seek serotonin when we're anxious, stressed out, or unhappy as it helps to regulate mood.

Low levels of serotonin have been linked to sugar cravings, as well as a variety of other symptoms like mood disorders, anxiety, and sleep disturbances. Serotonin is a neurotransmitter that is known to regulate mood, emotions of overall well-being, and hunger as well as food consumption.

Regular exercise is one strategy, which has been shown to elevate mood and lessen stress. soliciting assistance from close friends, family, or a mental health professional can be helpful for managing anxiety and stress and lowering the likelihood of engaging in unhealthy behaviors like overeating. Meditation and deep breathing exercises can also be helpful for managing anxiety and stress and lowering the likelihood of engaging in unhealthy behaviors like overeating.

Lack of sleep is linked to excessive eating, especially of junk food, so if you haven't had a good night's sleep in a while, it may have contributed to your recent desire for sugar. Try to get about eight hours of sleep each night to lessen your tendency to overindulge in sweets.

Make an enjoyable nighttime routine a habit.

If you're still having trouble falling asleep or staying asleep, you may have insomnia; speak to your doctor who can refer you to a sleep specialist. Get regular exercise, but avoid it two to three hours before bedtime; avoid daytime naps longer than 20 minutes (especially those taken later in the day); try to wake up and go to bed at the same time every day; avoid using your phone an hour before bedtime.

Lack of Nutrients:

If you find yourself feeling dizzy without sugar or experiencing consistently strong cravings, it's time to consult a specialist as it might suggest a deeper nutritional problem. For example, acute and (apparently) uncontrollable sugar cravings may result from a blood-sugar imbalance, such as hypoglycemia.

For example, if your body doesn't get enough magnesium, it will struggle to bring energy into the cells and will crave sugar to help raise energy levels. However, before you jump to any conclusions, keep in mind that your body's lack of certain minerals, which are involved in controlling insulin levels, could also affect your craving for sweets.

Thankfully, there are many healthy snacks you may munch on when you start to crave sugar, such as fresh fruit, almonds, Greek yogurt, and dark chocolate.

Fresh fruit: Fruit naturally contains sugar, and it also contains fiber and minerals (hello, antioxidants). Fruit also contains sugar, so it helps satisfy cravings.

Nuts and seeds: Nuts and seeds are a fantastic source of extra protein, fiber, and healthy fats and can make you feel full.

Greek yogurt: Similar to nuts and seeds, Greek yogurt also helps you feel fuller for longer and is packed with nutrients including calcium, bacteria that are good for your digestive system, and vitamins.

Dark chocolate: "Dark chocolate contains antioxidants and other healthy ingredients, has less sugar than milk chocolate, and tastes delicious."

If you love chocolate, you don't have to give up your comfort food. If you absolutely must have chocolate, go for a dark variety that has at least 70% cocoa content.

Bring out some cheese and whole-grain crackers that haven't had their beneficial fibers removed from them; this snack combo has plenty of protein, healthy fats, and complex carbohydrates to satisfy hunger in a satisfying and tasty way.

Chapter 8

Amplify your output

Similar to how a car runs best with a full tank of gas, your body needs the right kind of fuel from food to function at its best. A mix of carbohydrates, proteins, fats, minerals, vitamins, and water will provide your body with what it needs.

These suggestions can assist you in organizing your pre-workout meals so that you can prevent low blood sugar, avoid feeling hungry while working out, and fuel your muscles for both training and competition.

Eat a larger meal that includes carbohydrates, protein, and fat if you have 4+ hours before commencing your workout; if you only have 2-3 hours, eat smaller "mini" meals that are rich in carbohydrates and moderate in protein. You should eat carbohydrates at every meal and snack since they provide you with energy. It is preferable to eat whole-grain carbohydrates after your workout because they will provide you with sustained energy.

all great sources of complex carbohydrates. For quick energy, eat refined carbohydrates (such as white bread, white rice, and white crackers) for 30 to 60 minutes before going out.

Before heading out, avoid eating meals that are bulky or high in fiber, including broccoli, baked beans, or high-fiber cereal. Certain meals may give you stomachaches when you exercise because they digest more slowly. Be sure to have high-fiber meals throughout the rest of the day as well since they are rich in beneficial nutrients.

You shouldn't use sugars and sweets as fuel for exercise because they don't give you long-lasting energy, especially soda and candy.

Try to stay away from high-dietary-fat foods like fast food, ice cream, almonds, and cheese for your pre-workout lunch. Since they take a while to digest, if you eat a lot of these things right before going out, you can feel lethargic and exhausted.

Do not try new foods before a competition. You might have trouble digesting a new dish. Choose foods you are accustomed to eating on a training day or try something new.

Consume fresh or dry fruit, crackers, granola, cereal bars, pretzels, and applesauce 30 to 60 minutes before going out.

If you're exercising for longer than 90 minutes, sip water and Gatorade.

Two to three hours before leaving for the evening, have a granola bar and yogurt, a half-baguette or an English muffin with peanut butter and/or jelly, cereal and milk, or oatmeal with berries.

Ingest: water

Over four hours before your workout

Eat a balanced lunch that contains protein, good fats, and carbohydrates (grains with fruit or vegetables). An example of such a meal would be a turkey and cheese sandwich on wheat bread with lettuce and tomato, a piece of fruit, and a cup of pretzels.

Brown rice is served with grilled chicken, sweet potato, and vegetables.

A piece of fruit and an egg with cheese on a whole wheat bagel or English muffin. cereal in a bowl with milk, eggs, and fruit.

Depending on how long your workout is, you might or might not need to eat while exercising. Consider consuming something easy to digest that will provide you immediate energy, such as fruit, an energy bar, or pretzels, if your workout is taking more than an hour and a half. Consult a licensed nutritionist to see whether products like sports chews and gels designed for endurance athletes are appropriate for your level of exercise.

after an exercise: It's important to refuel your body following a demanding workout. It's important to eat some carbohydrates and protein as soon as possible after working out since your body requires time to rebuild muscle glycogen stores.

When planning your post-workout meal, keep the following in mind:

Even though people should eat after exercising, sometimes exercise might help people feel less hungry. Try consuming a snack with both protein and carbohydrates within 30-45 minutes of exercising, such as yogurt, a half-sandwich, or chocolate milk. Your body will heal more quickly as a result.

In the following two to three hours, you should have a larger meal that is high in carbs and contains protein to restore muscle glycogen stores and repair muscle tissues. You'll recover more quickly and be ready for your next workout if you do this.

How do I know I'm getting enough calories?

Your body needs calories to fuel exercise and replace any energy that is expended while participating in physical activity. If you cut calories, you can't perform at your best. The energy needs of exercise and athletic training, which exceed your body's everyday requirements, must be met in order to perform at your best and recover quickly after a session. If you skip meals, it will show in your performance. Regular meals and healthful snacks are the best way to fuel your body for sporting activity.

Since different foods have different levels of nutrients, you should eat a variety of meals in order to get all the nutrients you require to be in top shape. For instance, oranges lack iron and protein but are high in carbohydrates and vitamin C. Grilled chicken has iron and protein, but neither vitamin C nor carbohydrates. Always strive for a balance of carbohydrates, proteins, fats, minerals, vitamins, and water to operate at your peak.

Because they supply the body with the glucose it needs for energy (found in meals like pasta, bread, cereal, rice, cereals, potatoes, fruit, vegetables, milk, yogurt, etc.), carbohydrates, sometimes referred to as "carbs," are especially important for sports. Glycogen, your body's energy reserve, is stored as excess glucose in the liver and muscles. In order to maintain blood sugar levels and energy during brief bouts of exercise like running, basketball, gymnastics, or soccer, your body consumes glycogen. If you don't have enough glycogen, you can become extremely fatigued or find it difficult to continue the workout, which will undoubtedly impair how well you do. During extended exercise, your body mostly uses its glycogen stores to fuel performance, though depending on how long the activity lasts, it may also consume body fat reserves.

A large amount of fat is needed as fuel for longer activities and endurance sports like swimming, cycling, long-distance running, and hiking. Lack of dietary fat can affect athletic performance and cause other health problems, such as vitamin deficiencies because some vitamins require fat to be absorbed. Healthy sources of fat include avocados, salmon, nuts and nut butter, olive oils, and salmon.

To build and repair muscles, your body requires protein. Energy can occasionally be obtained from protein. Protein can be found in lean meats like chicken and turkey, beans, tofu, eggs, and dairy products like Greek yogurt, cheese, and milk.

Although they are not energy-producing substances, vitamins and minerals play a number of significant roles in the body. For instance, calcium and vitamin D are needed for strong bones, while iron and calcium are needed for blood cells to carry oxygen throughout the body. Specific minerals like sodium, calcium, and potassium are known as electrolytes. Since they have an effect on your body's water balance and muscular performance, they are essential during exercise. A balanced diet with a variety of foods should be consumed by athletes to ensure that they get enough vitamins and minerals. Regular multivitamins are fine, but supplements with a lot of vitamins and minerals don't help you perform better and might even be harmful. Consult your doctor or nutritionist if you believe your diet necessitates additional specialist supplements, such as iron, calcium/vitamin D, or B vitamins.

To stay hydrated, you must consume water. The symptoms of dehydration, which happen when your body doesn't have enough fluids to function correctly, include cramping in the muscles, fainting, and dizziness. While you are engaged in physical activity, dehydration is not only dangerous but can also impair your performance. Keep a water bottle nearby and sip from it periodically during the day to stay hydrated.

What is meant by "carb loading"?

Carbohydrate loading is a technique that can raise muscle glycogen stores. In the week before a competition, you eat more carbohydrates while doing fewer exercises. Carbohydrate loading is only necessary for marathon runners and other elite endurance athletes; it is not necessary for most sports.

Should I take supplements or eat extra protein?

Although some extra protein is needed to bulk up, most people get plenty through their meals. Increasing your protein intake won't provide any further advantages. In actuality, consuming enough calories—particularly from carbohydrates—is more important for muscle building than increasing protein intake. If you don't get enough calories, your body won't be able to build new muscle

Do I have to eat energy bars?

It differs. Energy bars come in many different varieties. While others may be heavy in protein, carbohydrates, or both, some may also be high in sugar. Although they don't contain any unique elements that can enhance your athletic performance, they are convenient and practical for travel and may make it simpler for you to fit a snack into a busy schedule. Foods like yogurt, cheese and crackers, or peanut butter and fruit are a few examples that are frequently less expensive and just as tasty (if not better) than energy snacks.

What types of water you should be drinking, and how much?

Athletes need more water since they sweat more than non-athletes do while exercising. It is not a good idea to wait until you are thirsty before you start drinking water because this indicates that you are starting to become dehydrated. Remember to drink even more when the weather is hot and sticky.

Drinking water prior to exercise tries to keep you properly hydrated before indulging in physical activity. Different people need different amounts of water before exercising depending on a variety of factors, including weight/height, how much they sweat before exercising, how much they've eaten, and the weather outside. Teenagers should typically drink 16 to 20 ounces (2 to 2.5 cups) of liquid at least two to three hours prior to engaging in physical activity, followed by 8 to 10 ounces (1 to 1.5 cups) of water 10 to 20 minutes prior to the exercise.

When exercising: How much fluid you need varies on your activity's intensity and duration, the surrounding conditions, and how much you perspire. It is recommended that you drink 12 to 1 cup (4 to 8 ounces) of liquids every 15-20 minutes while you are training (approximately 1 gulp of water equals 1 ounce). If you intend to exercise hard for more than 90 minutes, it may be good to take electrolyte-fortified water or a sports drink to replenish the electrolytes lost through perspiration.

after a workout: Calorie-dense liquids (such as milk, juice, or a sports drink) can take the place of water and glucose. Milk protein will help muscles repair and grow again. Your level of hydration can be assessed based on the color of your urine. An extremely light yellow tinge that is still transparent is a sign of good hydration. However, you should drink more fluids if you notice a more intense yellow tint. You should make an effort to replace lost fluids (between 16 and 24 ounces, or 2-3 cups) within the first two hours after ending an exercise session in order to rehydrate.

Should I drink sports drinks?

The best beverage to drink before, during, and after exercise is typically water. Electrolytes, water, and carbs are replaced with sports drinks like Gatorade® or Powerade®. It might be advantageous to have an energy drink if you're engaged in a strenuous sport. If you are exercising for longer than 90 minutes, unless you are exercising vigorously or in the heat, water is likely the best source of hydration.

Athletes need more calories and water than non-athletes, so keep that in mind. Regular meals and wholesome snacks are beneficial for your body before and after exercise. It's essential to give your body enough of the right nutrients in order to feel well and have the energy it needs to function at its best.

Chapter 9

The Science of Personal Change and Growth,

In the corporate world, paradigm shifts are commonplace and change is the only constant. A few examples are the transformation of analog to digital, spoken word to text, scheduled media to social media, etc. It is critical for people and businesses to understand how to effectively harness change for their benefit in the present business environment. In fact, there is a science of transition, a recently created field of research that looks into the human side of how people undergo significant, paradigm-shifting change. Transformational

Change frequently behaves nonlinearly and in ways that surprise us with their apparent suddenness, both on a personal and social level.

Transformational Principles
Understanding the following tips transformative principles is crucial for applying transformation science to organizational success:

Human brains are designed for change.
Tipping points, which are sudden changes that occur when a critical ratio is achieved, are the processes by which transformative change takes place.

Promises, which are a statement of will and dedication, can spur meaningful transformation.

It takes a deliberate way to transform.
Because the human brain is an organ that is always developing, we are not necessarily confined by our patterns of mental functioning. We have the capacity to alter our thinking, and this is not just a wish or a promise of psychotherapy; it is an instantaneously evident truth of the nature of our brains. The inherent ability of "neuroplasticity" to change regularly won't, however, happen on its own. We must deliberately take this possibility into account.

the capacity to radically alter your life through exercise.
While there are many methods to reach these goals—a complete life filled with achievement, pleasure, and health—regular exercise and physical fitness are among the most powerful and transformative approaches.

Our bodies produce endorphins during exercise, which are natural mood enhancers that help us fight against negative moods and emotions. Additionally, exercising gives us a constructive way to release stress and anxiety, which helps us feel more at ease and focused. Regular exercise has been shown to improve our mood, lower stress and anxiety levels, as well as lessen depressive symptoms.

Keeping a regular exercise schedule lowers our risk of developing chronic illnesses like heart disease, diabetes, and some types of cancer. It also strengthens our immune system, which can help us more successfully fight off infections and illnesses. Exercise also has a long-term impact on our general health and quality of life.

In addition to the physical and mental benefits, regular exercise may have a significant impact on our performance on a personal and professional level. We have more confidence in our abilities and strength when we feel strong and healthy, which may result in better professional performance, more solid interpersonal relationships, and a higher sense of self-worth.

We develop our capacity to push ourselves to our limits and overcome obstacles by creating and completing fitness objectives. These capacities may be applied in various facets of our lives, enabling us to fulfill our potential and accomplish our goals. Exercise can also help in the development of virtues like self-control, persistence, and resilience.

In conclusion, it's critical to recognize the power of fitness, as it has the power to positively impact a variety of aspects of our lives, from our physical and mental health to our capacity for success in both our personal and professional lives. If you haven't already, it's time to start prioritizing your fitness in order to enjoy its wonderful benefits.

Acknowledgments:

It is my sincere hope that the words in this book will give you the inspiration, optimism, and skills you need to transform your life for the better. As I come to the end of this life-changing trip known as "Fix Your Fitness," I want to express my sincere gratitude to all of the readers who have joined me on this journey. We are humbled by your confidence and openness to discovering new possibilities.

May "Fix Your Fitness" function as a catalyst for positive change, guiding you toward a life of wonderful health, fortitude, and self-discovery. Finally, I would want to express how pleased and honored I am to have had the opportunity to develop "Fix Your Fitness."

with the highest regard,

(Norman G. Johns)